Breath, Mind, and Consciousness

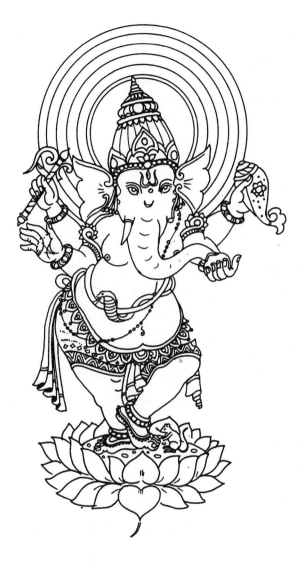

GANESHA MANTRA

गजाननम् भुत गणादि सेवितम्

कपित्य्य जम्बू फल चारु भक्षणम्

उमा सुतम् शोक विनाशकारकम्

नमामि विघ्नेश्वर पाद पंकजम्

Breath, Mind, and Consciousness

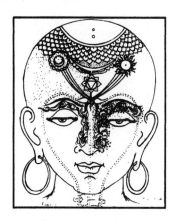

HARISH JOHARI

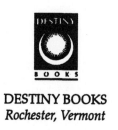

DESTINY BOOKS
Rochester, Vermont

Destiny Books
One Park Street
Rochester, Vermont 05767
www.gotoit.com

LIBRARY OF CONGRESS CATALOGING-IN-PUBLICATION DATA

Johari, Harish, 1934-
    Breath, mind, and consciousness / by Harish Johari.
       p. cm.
    Includes index.
    ISBN 978-0-89281-252-3
    1. Yoga. I. Title.
  BL1238.54.J64   1989
  181'.45—dc19 88-35175
       CIP

Printed and bound in the United States

10

Text design by Dede Cummings, Irving Perkins Associates.
This book was typeset in Garamond

Destiny Books is a division of Inner Traditions International

CONTENTS

ACKNOWLEDGMENTS

I AM INDEBTED to Baba Kailash Giri of Chaudhry Talab Temple, Bareilly, for introducing me to the wisdom of Swara Yoga. I thank Baba Santosh Dass and Baba Dwarika Dass, whose company gave me a clearer perspective on this science. Without good company—*satsang*—true understanding is impossible; it brings positive feedback, impetus, and the inspiration required to make progress in any branch of learning. Shyam Lal, the cobbler, Pandey Jo, Premji, and all my friends who practice Swara Yoga deserve thanks. In their company I was able to verify my tests of Swara Yoga while in India during 1965 and 1966.

As well I am grateful to Dr. Philip Epstein who helped me understand the relationship of Swara Yoga to neurobiology and neurochemistry. Dr. James Daley deserves special appreciation for introducing me to the Western vision of this yogic science. He was kind enough to provide me with a brain wave analyzer during my research in Oakland in 1972. I would also like to thank Dr. Shannahoff-Khalsa for his contribution to better mental health through an understanding of the relationship between the nostrils and the hemispheres of the brain.

Finally, I thank all my friends and students who have applied the knowledge of Swara Yoga and have made use of the Prana Calendar since I published the first edition in 1974. Carmen Carrero and Heidi Rauhut also deserve thanks for preparing the typed manuscript from my hand-written pages.

HARISH JOHARI
Uttar Pradesh
March, 1989

INTRODUCTION

BREATH IS the physical counterpart of the mind. The mind uses the cerebral cortex of the brain, the twin hemispheres, as its tool. These two hemispheres coordinate with the entire organism through neuromotor responses. All neuromotor activities, all sensory and motor functions of the body, are performed with the help of the breath. So breath is mind in action! Breath provides the pranic force to the organism. This pranic force, working as the Air element, creates movement, pulsation, vibration, and life. The word "spirit" comes from the Latin word *spiritus,* which literally means breath.

Mind and consciousness are abstract terms—whereas breath is a physiological reality. The study of consciousness begins with the study of the true science of breathing. Breath induces movement. Breathing itself is a neuromotor activity. The science of controlling prana is known as *pranayama,* a branch of Hatha Yoga. The term Yoga, which literally means union, refers to a discipline, a way of evolving the higher faculties of mind. There are many paths in Yoga, but in essence they all have one goal—the union of the self with God. On the physical level, this means the union of the lower brain with the upper brain. Man's faculties of abstract thinking and his aspirations for the higher ideals of life (seated in the cerebral cortex) often conflict with his instinctive, animal nature (seated in the lower brain). Through Yoga, man can learn to master his lower brain and pursue higher ideals, to act in accord with the law of universal good. While his animalistic nature makes man hedonistic and selfish, yogic training makes him selfless.

All yogic disciplines clearly state that a direct relationship exists between prana and mind and that by controlling or mastering prana one can master the mind. According to *Yoga Kundalyupanishad,* the breathing process creates images in the mind; by controlling the breathing process through pranayama, the breath becomes calm, images do not disturb the mind, and the internal dialogue stops. According to Dr. David Shannahoff-Khalsa of the Salk Institute for Biological Studies in San Diego, "The nose is an instrument for altering cortical activity." (See Figure 1.) Stop the prana and mental modifications will stop, and the yogi will be able to establish himself in bliss (*samadhi*). Prana refers not only to the flow of oxygen into the organism but to all components of life force. Prana is the vital life force that sustains all living organisms. Pranic energy is available in negative ions, oxygen, ozone, and solar radiation, but for human beings its main source is the breath.

Swara Yoga is the science of nasal breath. It has rightly been called the "ancient technology of mind."* Not a

*The words of Dr. Shannahoff-Khalsa taken from *Brain Mind Bulletin,* Vol. 8, No. 3, Jan. 3, 1983.

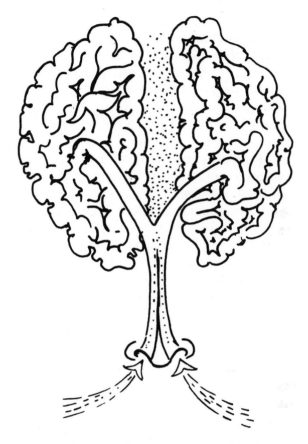

FIGURE 1. Posterior view of the hemispheres of the brain and their relationship to the respiratory system. Breath coming in through the right nostril cools the right hemisphere of the brain, causing the left hemisphere to become active. Breath coming in through the left nostril has the opposite effect.

part of Hatha Yoga or other yogas, the science of Swara Yoga deals with the relationship between the nasal breath and the subtle nerves of the body, on the one hand, and the cycles of the Moon and the elements, on the other. It studies the nasal cycles—the nature of the breath flowing with the right and left nostrils. The teachings of Swara Yoga allow us to synchronize our breath, our life, with the universal rhythm of the Moon. This alignment removes the effort and strain from our daily activities and brings good fortune.

The founders of Swara Yoga were not familiar with the cerebral hemispheres, but they did work with the principle of bipolarity: the right side of the body being the masculine, solar principle, or Shiva, and the left being the feminine, lunar principle, or Shakti. Reaching into the depths of human behavior, they were able to ascertain which activities were best suited for right nasal dominance, and which for left. By observing the direct effect of the moon on the breath, they discovered the sacred science of right living. This book offers methods for determining right/left nostril dominance and for synchronizing the dominant nostril with specific activities of everyday life.

"The implication of this technology is that we are not helpless victims of a given emotional state. 'If you want to alter an unwanted state,' says Dr. Shannahoff-Khalsa, 'just breathe through the more congested nostril.' "* By altering the flow of nasal breath, the body chemistry gradually changes, and unwanted emotional and physiological states slowly disappear.

Swara Yoga can teach human beings the precise way of living peacefully, as masters of their own mind and body; it can enable them to become true instruments of Consciousness. This book gives the reader a key for "self-tuning the body/mind with the body/mind itself as the tuning instrument."**

----

*The words of Dr. Shannahoff-Khalsa taken from *Brain Mind Bulletin,* Vol. 8, No. 3, Jan. 3, 1983.

**Quote from John Lynch, *Brain Mind Bulletin,* Vol. 8, No. 3, January, 1983, p.3.

CHAPTER 1

The Science of Swara Yoga

OUR HUMAN ORGANISM works through a specialized network of channels known to physical science as nerves, veins, and arteries. Those conduits that enable us to act and react to our environment are known as nerves. We will use the term *nadi* to refer to the subtle nerves of the body. The autonomic nervous system runs the inner machinery of the organism via the sympathic and parasympathetic branches. All nerves and nadis form a network around each cell, fiber, tissue, bone, etc., to keep the organism conscious of its environment and itself. As long as the flow of energy in each nadi and nerve is working in proper rhythmic order in a particular area, life exists. When the nadis are blocked, the organ connected with them becomes lifeless, and as a result the organism develops many diseases.

Our internal organs function much like a factory, producing energy that gets converted into consciousness.

The cerebral cortex receives neuromotor signals from the internal organs in the form of electrical impulses which are then interpreted and converted into consciousness. These neuromotor signals themselves take the form of electromagnetic and electrochemical energy. The "manufacturing" process continues as long as one is breathing, except during yogic breathing when the process is sustained in the absence of ordinary breathing. When breath stops altogether the organism dies. Breath is the very key to life. It connects the organism with consciousness, matter with mind. Its presence is life and absence, death.

Breath is prana, but the breathing process itself is a neuromotor action since inhalation and exhalation are done with the help of the nerves. This action is produced by the pulsation of life. Action is needed for all cell division. According to Indian philosophy, this action exists in the very seed of the organism as a function of the Wind element. Pulsation, contraction, expansion, and breathing are actions inherent to the sperm and ovum. It is this inherent throbbing or pulsation that sustains the organism before its first breath occurs. Even when the nostrils are not operative and the lungs are dormant, amniotic fluid, charged with pranic ions from the mother, flows into the lungs and through the umbilical cord; thus prana functions inside the womb. After fertilization, growth starts; the pranic force needed for this growth is provided inside the womb where the organism is perfectly sealed and nourished by the fluids of life. After birth, the first thing that regulates all bodily activity is breath—the expansion of the lungs and opening of the nostrils. The lungs begin to operate with the first cry of the baby. This is the starting point of individual life, and of the nasal cycle.

Proper Breathing and Its Effects on Life Span

The nose is the only bodily organ in continuous interplay with the external environment. The rate of our breathing quickly responds to changes in our physical or mental condition. In anger, for example, breathing becomes fast, and during deep sleep it becomes slow and regular. An average human organism breathes (one inhale and one exhale) thirteen to fifteen times a minute, which means that our body breathes 21,000 to 21,600 times in a twenty-four-hour cycle. With an increase in the rhythm of breathing comes an increase in the flow of blood and other vital life fluids. These increases in turn stimulate neuromotor activity that causes the body to utilize more energy. The organism then must convert more oxygen and glucose into energy through internal cellular respiration. These demands do not affect the organism in its growing cycle, but in maturity the organism reacts to wear and tear, the repair mechanism slows down, and the energy level is reduced. The result is increased stress and strain. By maintaining a normal breathing rate of not more than fifteen breaths per minute, or by slowing down the breathing rate, we can conserve energy, increase our level of vitality, and live longer.

According to the scriptures of Swara Yoga, *Shiva Swarodaya* and *Gyana Swarodaya,** the life span of a man is measured not in years but in number of breaths. At the rate of fifteen breaths per minute, a human life is comprised of a total of 946,080,000 breaths—a full 120 years. To maintain the normal breathing rate, i.e., fifteen

Gyana Swarodaya has not yet been translated into English. The Sanskrit text of *Shiva Swarodaya,* with an English translation by Ram Kumar Rai, has been published by Prachya Prakashan, Varanasi 74, A Jagatganj, Varanasi 221002, U.P. India.

breaths per minute, does not call for special effort or training. Slowing down the breathing rate, however, requires control over the breathing process and diligent practice of pranayama. Swara Yoga also prescribes methods of controlling breath by the power of will. One practice, for example, involves slowing down the breathing rate by concentration on the sound of the inhaling breath and the exhaling breath. In normal breathing there is no audible sound, but when one breathes fast the sound becomes more and more pronounced. When this happens, one should try to overcome the fast breathing by concentrating on the sound of the breath and slowing down the activity in the body. During normal breathing, one complete breath takes four seconds and the exhaled breath extends the distance of twelve finger widths. As one reduces the rate of breathing, one automatically reduces the length (in distance) of breath. By reducing the length of the breath and simultaneously the breath rate, one's life span increases.

Nostrils and the Brain

Each nostril, when it operates independently, influences the body chemistry in a different way. When both nostrils operate simultaneously, the body chemistry alters so as to make meditation rather than worldly activity appropriate to engage in. The right nostril, being solar or heating in character, increases acidic secretions, whereas the left nostril, being lunar or cooling, increases alkaline secretions. Both right and left nostrils are connected with the opposite sides of the cerebral hemispheres and the olfactory lobe. Since the alternation of breath from one nostril to the other is regulated directly by opposing sympathetic and parasympathetic commands,* it is possible that the hypothalamus is the center of the mental processes and behavior in humans. The nose is in direct contact with the hypothalamus by its link with the olfactory lobe of the brain. The hypothalamus regulates body temperature, which influences the mental processes that are interpreted by the brain as emotional states. The hypothalamus is a part of the limbic system—that part of the brain associated with emotions and motivation.

Nostrils, by means of the process of respiration, are connected with neuromotor responses and thus with the autonomic nervous system (sympathetic and parasympathetic). These neuromotor responses influence the hemispheres of the brain and the primary activity of the brain, which is chemical. Neurotransmitters are the brain's chemical messengers; they influence all body functions, including temperature, blood pressure, hormone levels, and regular circadian rhythms.

NATURE OF THE NOSTRILS

Through a network of sensory nerves in the nose, the nostrils are connected to subtle nerves, or nadis. These nadis are of two kinds:

1. Conduits of pranic force—*pranavaha nadi*
2. Conduits of psychic energy—*manovaha nadi*

Some of the most important nadis carry both pranic energy (flowing as electromagnetic currents) and psychic

---

*The sympathetic nervous system is more active during the flow of breath through *Pingala,* the solar nadi; the parasympathetic nervous system is more active during the flow of breath through *Ida,* the lunar nadi.

energy (flowing as feeling, vibrations, frequencies, etc.) at the same time.

Yogic texts mention fourteen important nadis that carry both kinds of energy. Three of these fourteen are of vital importance. These three nadis, Ida, Pingala and Sushumna, are connected with the limbic system. Activating Ida influences the hypothalamus and the pituitary gland, and thus the growth hormones and anabolic processes; activating Pingala influences the thalamus and hypothalamus but not the pituitary. The Sushumna is connected with the corpus callosum and the cerebellum. When it bifurcates in the brain stem, one branch of the Sushumna goes to the corpus callosum, while the other, known as the posterior Sushumna, passes through the cerebellum to the cerebral cortex and terminates in the corpus callosum. Here it joins the other branch, known as the anterior Sushumna. This point of termination is called the fontanella (the "soft spot" in an infant's skull that hardens after three to six months). (See Figures 2 and 3 for a further look at the human brain.) Through their connection with the endocrine glands, these three nadis influence body chemistry and the chemical nature of the human organism. The Sushumna nadi is the only nadi that directly pierces all the chakras or psychic centers of the subtle body. These centers are connected with internal organs through sympathetic and parasympathetic nerves, which are connected with the autonomic nervous system working through the spinal column. The Sushumna is thus connected with the network of sympathetic and parasympathetic nerves and the autonomic nervous system through its connection to the chakras and its passage through the spinal column. Although the three nadis meet at the same place in the pelvic plexus, they originate in different parts of the *Muladhara,* or the base of the spine (see *Chakras,* * pp. 20–28).

*Harish Johari, *Chakras* (Rochester, Vermont: Destiny Books, 1987).

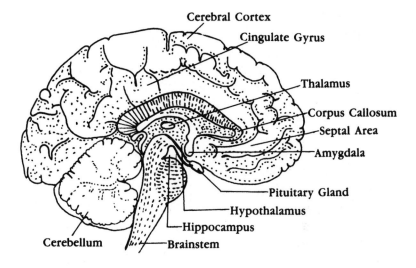

FIGURE 2. Cross-section of the human brain showing the limbic system.

Ida and Pingala are located on the left and right side of the spine respectively, but when they are activated, through yogic breathing (pranayama) and the movement of the activated spiritual energy or Kundalini, they criss-cross as they move and work on the first five chakras. While the Sushumna terminates in the crown chakra or Sahasrara, the Ida and Pingala nadis terminate in the left and right nostril respectively (see Figure 4). The passage of the Sushumna opens only with awakening of the Kundalini which, when dormant, resides in the Muladhara or root chakra. Once activated, this Kundalini energy travels up the body through a very fine channel called *brahmanadi,* located within the Sushumna.

1. **Ida:** This nadi originates at the base of the spine (Muladhara) and works as the left channel. It flows on the left side of the spinal column and terminates in the left nostril by branching into fine capillaries. This nadi becomes active when breathing is carried out by

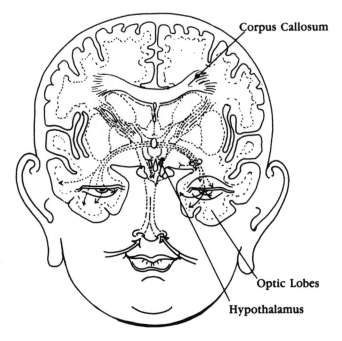

Corpus Callosum

Optic Lobes

Hypothalamus

FIGURE 3. Front view of the brain showing the hypothalamus.

the left nostril. Since Ida is considered to be nourishing and purifying, its energy is called feminine or maternal. The left nostril is connected with the right cerebral hemisphere, making it emotional and magnetic in nature. Because of its dominance during the ascending cycle of the Moon, it is called lunar. The breath flowing through the left nostril is called Ida, or Moon breath.

2. **Pingala:** This nadi originates at the base of the spine and acts as the right channel. It is situated on the right side of the spinal column and terminates in the right nostril, also by branching into fine capillaries. During the operation of the right nostril this nadi becomes active. It is connected with solar currents and its

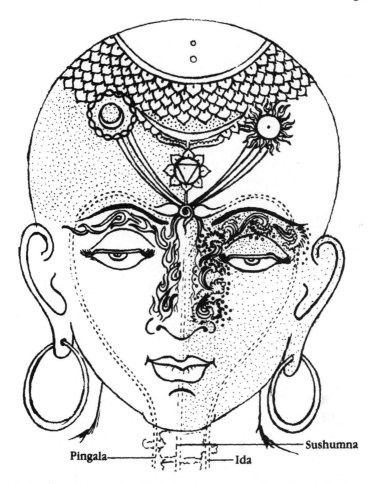

FIGURE 4.   Ida (lunar) and Pingala (solar) nadis terminating in left
and right nostrils. Energies cross at area of third eye.

energy is considered to be masculine. The right nostril is connected with the left cerebral hemisphere,
making it verbal and rational in nature. Because it is
dominant during the descending cycle of the Moon, it
is called solar. The breath flowing through the right
nostil is called Pingala, or Sun breath.

3. **Sushumna:** This nadi originates at the base of the spine and is situated between the Ida and Pingala. It is also known as the central canal or the royal way. Its energy flows through the interior of the spinal column. It pierces the palate at the base of the skull and terminates at the top of the skull.

When air flows in both nostrils equally, the Sushumna nadi becomes active. It is fiery in nature. This nadi usually works at dawn or dusk automatically and also, for short intervals, when the transition from one nostril to the other nostril takes place. All human beings breathe through both nostrils just before death, when Sushumna becomes active.

Thus, we see the nostrils are named after their relationship with the solar and lunar currents, which are respectively heating and cooling in nature. Through the periodic alternation of the nostrils the chemical balance is maintained within the organism.

Nostrils and the Planets

The relationship between the nostrils and the lunar cycles has not yet been discovered by Western neurophysiologists. However Swara Yoga, as documented by the scripture *Shiva Swarodaya,* has known about this relationship since ancient times. These yogis have clearly stated:

1. The right nostril, which is masculine and connected with the left hemisphere, is associated with the solar planets: the Sun, Mars, and Saturn. On the days corresponding to these planets—Sunday, Tuesday and Saturday—the right nostril works for one hour, starting ninety minutes before sunrise. Half an hour before

sunrise, it changes and the nostril of the day (see section that follows) takes over. When the right nostril is also the nostril of the day, flow of breath through this nostril on these three days is auspicious.

2. The left nostril, which is feminine and connected with the right hemisphere, is associated with the lunar planets: the Moon, Mercury, Jupiter and Venus. Every Monday, Wednesday, Thursday, and Friday the left nostril works for one hour, starting ninety minutes before sunrise. Half an hour before sunrise, the nostril of the day takes over. When the left nostril is also the nostril of the day, flow of breath through this nostril on these four days is auspicious.

3. The Sushumna nadi is active when both nostrils function together. It automatically operates very briefly at dawn or dusk, when the nostril connected with the planet (as described above) stops and the nostril of the day takes over. This nadi is not influenced by either the ascending and descending cycles of the moon.

Nostrils and the Moon

To synchronize the breath with the lunar rhythm is to align oneself with a profound life-giving energy. The moon is not just a mass of matter floating in space; it influences the fluids in the body, which form the essence of our body chemistry. Moon cycles also affect moods.*

The nostrils are directly related to the cycles of the moon. During the ascending and descending lunar cycles, the left and right nostrils are alternately dominant. For convenience, we count fifteen days in the ascending cycle and fifteen days in the descending cycle, making it a thirty-day cycle. But these are lunar days, not solar. The

*See *Brain Mind Bulletin*, May 20, 1984, Vol. 9, Number 10, p. 3.

moon takes only twenty-eight and a half days to complete its one revolution around the Earth. Our understanding of a day is based on the twenty-four-hour cycle in which the Earth completes one rotation on its axis. The different speeds of Earth and Moon create a complicated pattern. Not every moon date corresponds with the sunrise point on which our dates are based. For this reason, one should consult a Prana Calendar.*

In the ascending moon cycle, the left nostril operates for nine days, on lunar dates 1, 2, 3, 7, 8, 9, 13, 14, 15. In the same cycle, the right nostril operates for six days, on lunar dates 4, 5, 6, 10, 11, 12.

In the descending moon cycle, the right nostril likewise operates for nine days, on lunar dates 1, 2, 3, 7, 8, 9, 13, 14, 15. In the same cycle, the left nostril operates for six days, on lunar dates 4, 5, 6, 10, 11, 12. The right nostril operates for nine days and the left for six days.

The same nostril that starts the day one hour before sunrise also ends the day, at sunset.

Bimonthly Nostril Check

The moon changes bimonthly, or twice a month, creating two cycles:

1. Ascending cycle (from new moon to full moon) when the moon is gradually increasing in size and influence.
2. Descending cycle (from full moon to new moon) when the moon is gradually decreasing in size and affect.

*To order a Prana Calendar, write to Sri Center International, P.O. Box 2927, Rockefeller Center Station, NY, NY 10185.

As mentioned above, the left nostril dominates in the ascending lunar cycle and the right nostril in the descending cycle. If the Prana Calendar is not available, it is easy to find out if one is flowing with the lunar rhythm or not. To do so, one has simply to note the dominance of one's nostril at dawn following the full moon and new moon nights.

The morning following the full moon, the descending moon cycle starts; at dawn, the right nostril should operate for three consecutive days.

The morning following the new moon, the ascending moon cycle starts; at dawn, the left nostril should operate for three consecutive days.

If the nostrils are working properly, the body maintains its natural, healthful rhythm. If the correct nostril (right, following the full moon night and left, following the new moon night) is not working, there will be a change in one's body chemistry. This alteration can lead to physiological or psychological problems, or both, within that two-week period. It is therefore important to try to correct the problem at the outset. The nostrils should be checked around dawn before getting out of bed. In the event of wrong nostril dominance, one should not leave bed until the correct nostril starts operating. One should wait approximately ten to thirty minutes after sunrise and then change nostrils by forced breathing through the congested nostril. Other techniques mentioned in the section "How to Change the Nostril" may also be used. It is possible that the nostril of the day may start ten to thirty minutes before or after sunrise. Sometimes when the body chemistry is imbalanced the nostrils do not change, even after all methods have been tried. In such a case, one should become alert and act according to the operating nostril.

METHODS OF IDENTIFYING THE DOMINATING NOSTRIL

To determine which nostril is dominant one can:

1. Press one nostril and note if the breath is passing through the opposite nostril unobstructed. If not, press the congested nostril. Note that the dominant nostril will have an unobstructed flow of breath.
2. Breathe out quickly many times in a row without plugging either nostril; a cool sensation will be felt on the side of the open nostril.
3. Breathe out on a piece of glass or a mirror. The residual vapor deposit on the side of the operating nostril will be visually larger.

If the vapor desposit from both nostrils is of the same size, it indicates the working of both nostrils simultaneously. At these times, the Sushumna is dominant; both nostrils will breathe freely. There will be no obstruction on either side or equal obstruction on both sides will be felt.

HOW TO CHANGE THE NOSTRIL

When it is necessary to change the operating nostril, one can use any of the following three methods:

1. Lie down on the side of the operating nostril, e.g., on the right side when the right nostril is operating and vice versa. Place a small cushion under the armpit bearing the weight to stimulate the nerves on that side. The nostril should change within a few minutes. In healthy people, this position will cause the nostrils to change quickly—within two to three minutes. But when the body chemistry is imbalanced, the change takes longer. In the presence of illness, an hour may

not be enough to change the operating nostril; it could take as long as several hours.

2. Press the operating nostril gently with the thumb and breathe forcefully through the congested nostril.

3. Sit in a comfortable posture and turn the gaze toward the congested nostril. This practice can often be effectively combined with the forced breathing.

The first of these three methods, however, is the most effective and easiest for most people to practice. Lying on the side of the operating nostril provides relaxation and reduces anxiety. The nostril changes easily when one is relaxed; the force of gravity is also helpful. Practitioners of Swara Yoga, children, and persons with a pure body chemistry can change the breath of their nostrils in two to three minutes; Swara yogis can change it by will alone.

WHEN TO CHANGE THE NOSTRIL

It is important to change the operating nostril when any of the following circumstances prevail:

• If an activity needs to be done that does not correspond to the operating nostril (see Table 2 page 27).

• If one feels disturbed, show signs of an illness, experiences an unusual taste in the mouth, or a lack of energy.

• If the right or left nostril operates for more than two or three hours in a row.

• If the Moon nostril operates at the time the Sun nostril should naturally be operating, or vice versa.

• If both nostrils operate and something other than relaxation, meditation, or any act that can lead to realization needs to be done.

Incorrect operation of the nostrils creates tension and conflict, unnecessary activity, and loss. The nostrils should be changed whenever necessary.

Importance of the Nostrils

In Swara Yoga the nostrils serve as portals for respiration and indicators for the relative dominance of sympathetic and parasympathetic influences associated with the lateralization of activity in the twin hemishperes. They also serve as:

- A link connecting man and his environment;
- A connecting link between the physical body and the subtle bodies of man, matter with mind, energy with consciousness; and
- Indicators of coming events.

When the nostrils are perfectly synchronized with the solar and lunar rhythms, one can understand the subtle signals they give. The nostrils, through their link with the subtle bodies, can provide us with information about future events; by their abnormal behavior, they give clues to the organism about what is going to happen. Under normal conditions, the breath flows through one nostril for one to two hours, then alternates. When something significant is going to happen inside the organism, or outside in the environment, the breath flow starts behaving in an abnormal manner.

ABNORMALITIES IN THE NASAL CYCLES

- The nasal breaths do not alternate at regular intervals.
- Their synchronization with lunar rhythms (see page 15) is disrupted.

- The nasal breath that starts the day around sunrise is not also operating at the time of sunset, as it should.

- The nasal breaths alternate very quickly, breath does not take place through one nostril only, and both nostrils start working simultaneously at dawn.

When one starts practicing Swara Yoga, one becomes increasingly conscious of these abnormalities in the nasal cycle and their periodic alternation. The scriptures on Swara Yoga state that good as well as bad results are associated with the abnormal behavior of the nostrils. Change in duration of the left nostril normally brings good results; bad results are primarily the product of change in the duration of the right nostril, change in the joint operation of both nostrils, or when both nostrils alternate quickly.

Long duration of operation of the left nostril is usually beneficial. If the left nostril (Ida) operates:

- for more than two hours* in a row, the person will get something unexpected

- for more than three hours in a row, there will be unexpected gain

- for more than four hours, the person will get physical comforts, pleasure and peace

- for more than seven hours in a row, the person meets his or her beloved and makes new, beneficial friends

- for twenty-four hours in a row, the person obtains splendor, glory, and a raise in status and the luxuries of life.

*Note: Swara Yoga maintains that each nostril should operate for only one hour. However, some recent observations in the United States indicate that nostrils alternate on an average of every two to three hours. If this is true, the regular flow of the left nostril for more than three hours in a row will bring similar results.

If the left nostril operates during the day and the right nostril operates during the night every day, one lives up to 120 years in good mental and physical health.

If on the second day of the ascending cycle, the left nostril works at the time of the right nostril—that is, three hours after sunrise, when it should change to the right nostril—it is beneficial. Undertaking pious activities at such a time brings pleasure and benefit.

Long duration of the left nostril, however, can also be harmful. If the left nostril (Ida) operates:

- for five hours in a row, it indicates forthcoming physical ailment or pain in the body
- for six hours in a row, one has to face opposition, aggression, and obstructions
- for twenty-four hours in a row for a period of one, two or three days, one gets disease
- for five days in a row, one loses interest in the world outside and acquires emotional tension
- for one month continuously, one suffers loss of personal wealth and possessions

Long duration of the right nostril, except at night, brings bad results. If the right nostril (Pingala) operates:

- for more than two hours in a row, something valuable gets lost, or some kind of loss in wealth is indicated
- for more than three hours, one gets enmity with a good person
- for more than ten-and-one-half hours, one becomes aggressive, harsh, destructive and obnoxious
- for twenty-four hours in a row, one gets sick, decays slowly, and dies within three years

If both nostrils operate and alternate after half a day, one gets fame and earns good luck. When both nostrils operate simultaneously, Sushumna becomes dominant; actions taken at this time bring adverse results and unfavorable situations.

If both nostrils alternate very quickly, it indicates forthcoming troubles, failures, and obstacles.

One should always check the nostrils before:

- making decisions
- getting out of bed; leaving home, town, city or country
- entering any room, home, office, vehicle or country

If the left nostril is working, all movements of the lower body should be initiated with the left foot, and vice versa. That is, one should step out of bed by placing the left foot on the floor; one should leave a place (home, town, or country) by stepping out with the left foot; one should enter a new place (room, house, office, or vehicle) or enter a country by stepping in with the left foot first, and vice versa.

Before deciding to undertake an activity, one must consider the nature of the activity and whether or not the moment is right to act. Swara Yoga clearly states that certain activities are best performed when a particular nostril is operating (see Table 2, page 27). This information can be helpful in making decisions. Everyone can mark which nostril is operating when a particular thought or idea comes to mind. Nostril dominance can reveal whether or not the idea or thought will be beneficial, whether or not it will mature, and if the plans evolved from the ideas will succeed. If the day is solar (Sunday, Tuesday, or Saturday), started with the right (solar) nostril, and the idea, thought, or plan comes to mind while the right nostril is operating, one should pursue the matter. If, in addition, the activity is also connected with the right nostril, the idea, thought, or plan should be acted upon quickly.

The Nostrils and Special Activities

By direct observation, the Swara yogis discovered the link between breath and the efficient performance of specific activities. Their findings correspond to the observations of contemporary neurobiologists who have discovered that changes in cerebral dominance occasionally occur prior to changes in nostril dominance. Both ancient and modern scientists corroborate: the right side of the body is connected with the left hemisphere of the brain and vice versa (see Figure 5). Breath directly influences the peripheral autonomic nervous function. Breathing through the left nostril definitely influences the cortical activity on the right side of the brain more than the left, and vice versa. In the words of Dr. Khalsa, "Right nostril/left hemisphere dominance corresponds to phases of increased activity. Left nostril/right hemisphere dominance represents the rest phase."[*]

As mentioned earlier, breath is connected with the mind, which uses the brain as its tool. The twin hemispheres of the brain are tools of the mind, each with specific, highly specialized functions (although they do share some activities). This specialization is called lateralization of activity in the hemispheres. Localization of function, which is asymmetrical, makes the hemispheres have separate cognitive strategies. However, the brain-mind functions in a holographic manner to synthesize and integrate sensate responses, thinking, and higher intuition (perception) into a multidimensional awareness.

[*]See *Brain Mind Bulletin,* Vol. 8, No. 3, Jan. 3, 1983.

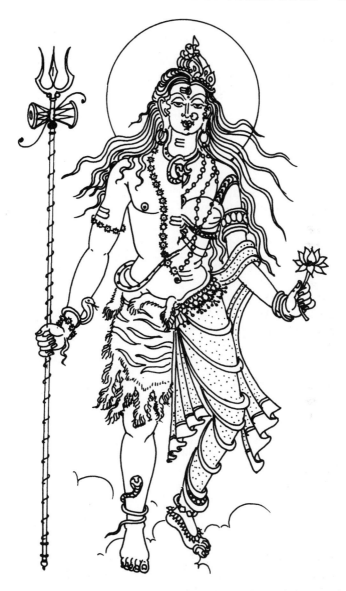

FIGURE 5.   The ancient concept of the right side of the body being
male (Shiva) and the left side being female (Shakti) can be
seen in this depiction of the Hindu deity Ardha Narish-
wara.

Under the dominance of different hemispheres, a person will handle the same situation in a different manner. The nostrils serve as indicators of cerebral dominance and may help the person anticipate his or her response to given circumstances. If one understands this point and performs those actions that are best suited for the hemisphere that is dominant at that moment, one can make the best use of his or her energy.

An effort should be made to undertake activities, either during the day or night, that are suitable to the dominant nostril.

Table 1. Qualities Associated with the Nostrils

LEFT NOSTRIL	RIGHT NOSTRIL
Days: Monday, Wednesday, Thursday, and Friday	*Days:* Sunday, Tuesday, Saturday
Cycle: Ascending Moon Cycle	*Cycle:* Descending Moon Cycle
Directions (to be avoided for travel): East and North*	*Directions* (to be avoided for travel): West and South*
*Influential Levels:** Ahead, left, above	*Influential levels:** Behind, right, below
Nature: Magnetic, feminine, lunar, alkaline	*Nature:* Electrical, masculine, solar, acidic
Suitable for: Peaceful activities	*Suitable for:* Difficult activities
Duration: One to two hours	*Duration:* One to two hours
Connected with: Right hemisphere of the brain; left side of the body	*Connected with:* Left hemisphere of the brain; right side of the body
Dominant: Morning following new moon night	*Dominant:* Morning following full moon night
Sanskrit Name: Ida	*Sanskrit Name:* Pingala
Body Chemistry: Mucus dominated	*Body Chemistry:* Bile dominated

* Facing these directions, however, during the performance of certain Tantric rituals brings beneficial results. See Johari's *Tools for Tantra* (Rochester, Vermont: Destiny Books, 1986), p. 62.

** Anyone positioned in these directions, in relation to your body, becomes subject to the influence of this nostril. In such a situation, gaining favors from the person or influencing his or her thoughts becomes easy.

Table 2. Activities Associated with the Nostrils*

LEFT NOSTRIL	RIGHT NOSTRIL
1. Stable business, requiring no movement	1. Unstable business, requiring movement
2. Long-term activities	2. Temporary activities or jobs that can be accomplished quickly
3. Journey to a far-off place	3. Journey to a near place
4. Collection of ornaments	4. Return journey
5. Collecting food grains and necessities of life	5. Studying or teaching martial arts
6. Beginning of study (regular school education)	6. Studying hard skills and destructive sciences
7. Playing musical instrument	7. Writing manuscripts
8. Singing	8. Practice of Shastras
9. Learning to dance	9. Practice of Tantra (yantra and mantra)
10. Construction of hermitage, temple	10. Destruction of country
11. Planting, gardening	11. Chopping wood, lighting a fire
12. Building wells, swimming pools, ponds	12. Cutting gems and jewels, sculpting, carpentry
13. Giving charity, lending money	13. Accepting charity, borrowing
14. Marriage; birth of baby	14. Prostitution, sexual indulgence (for male only)
15. Purchasing clothes, ornaments, and land	15. Selling cattle
16. Performing rituals for pacification, appeasement, and attaining worldly prosperity	16. Committing crimes; corrupt practices
17. Friendship; meeting relatives	17. Eradicating, poisoning, or subduing enemies
18. Making efforts to establish peace	18. Hunting, killing; holding a sword
19. Preparing divine medicine or chemicals; practice of alchemy	19. Practicing medicine
20. Treatment of diseases, therapy	20. Fighting, dueling, wrestling, boxing

(Continued)

*Note: The information given in Table 2 is very ancient. Although it attempts to span the entire panorama of human behavior, we can expand upon these lists by observing how modern-day activities fit into the specialized functions of the twin hemispheres.

Table 2. (Continued)

LEFT NOSTRIL	RIGHT NOSTRIL
21. Worshiping of the Guru	21. Seeing a king, meeting and addressing officials
22. Entering a newly constructed house, village, town, new country	22. Driving a vehicle
23. Thinking about relative's ill health	23. Having a discussion or debate
24. Being initiated into a spiritual order; practicing disciplines	24. Climbing a mountain
25. Addressing one's master	25. Invoking and mastering evil spirits; pacifying poison
26. Service	26. Ordering, giving commands
27. Performing auspicious acts	27. Gambling
28. Starting a new colony, order, or community	28. Swimming across a torrential river
29. Opening a bank account	29. Worshiping evil spirits, mastering mantra for power, vigor and bravery
30. Knowledge of past, present and future	30. Knowledge of unseen and unheard things
31. Curing fever	31. Purification by vomiting, enema, throat cleansing, water purification of the lower intestinal tract, sinus cleansing, Hatha Yoga exercise, *Kapal Bhati*
32. Applying sandalwood paste to the forehead	32. Using drugs and poisons
33. Tying a four-legged animal	33. Taming or riding a four-legged animal
34. Taking a new vow	34. Drinking liquor
35. Drinking non-alcholic beverages	35. Eating and defecating
36. Urinating	36. Bathing
37. Meditating	37. Captivating members of the opposite sex (for male only)
	38. Expressing anger
	39. Producing works of illumination
	40. Working with accounts, counting, preparing ledgers

SUSHUMNA ACTIVITIES

In Sushumna breathing, the nostrils operate jointly and airflow is bilaterally equal. Sushumna is also dominant when both nostrils alternate quickly.

Breathing through this nadi is poisonous; if both nostrils operate simultaneously for more than five hours in a row, it creates fatal illness. According to *Ayurveda* (Ayu = life; Veda = knowledge; Ayurveda = the science of right living)—the ancient Indian system of medicine in India—during Sushumna dominance the body chemistry is Wind dominated. This breath is meant only for calming the system and preparing it for a change in nostrils.

All plans made during Sushumna dominance fail, activities started remain incomplete, vows made at this time will be broken, and charity becomes useless.

The practice of fasting and meditation during Sushumna dominance gives complete absorption in the subtle source of all existence. Only centering the mind, meditating, observing silence, and chanting cures the poisons produced in the Sushumna.

Many of the psychological problems found in the West are due to left-hemisphere dominance. It is generally thought that people in the Western world are left-hemisphere dominated, whereas in tribal cultures, such as India and Africa, the people are more right-hemisphere oriented. Thus the problem of being dominated by one hemisphere exists in both East and West. It is a problem that can be easily solved by watching one's nostrils and regulating them periodically.

The information in Table 3, as revealed by modern science, was grasped intuitively by the Tantrics who, in ancient times, learned to work with the swara long ago. The aim of Swara Yoga was to educate man to (1) be relaxed and conscious of his own state of being before starting an activity, and (2) live in constant awareness of

Table 3. Behavior Associated with Right and Left Hemispheres*

LEFT HEMISPHERE	RIGHT HEMISPHERE
Speech, writing, and abstract power of conversation increases; vocabulary becomes richer and more varied	Nonverbal memory, emotional thinking and concrete thinking
Likes discussions	Sharply diminished capacity for speech
Answers questions in a more detailed, extensive manner	Difficulty in recalling names of objects in daily use, although the objects are recognized
Becomes excessively talkative	Uses short, simple sentences
Becomes more receptive to what others say	Speech activity is reduced
Is untouched by intonations of sound or emotions behind sounds	Answers are given by mime and gestures instead of words
Is unable to distinguish between male and female sounds	Difficulty in conversing
Is unable to pair patterns	Silence and inattentiveness to speech
Powers to grasp or recognize lessen	Hearing of loud sounds only; distinction between moods and intonations remains
Imagination and perception becomes defective	Can distinguish between male and female sounds
Long-term memory remains	Nonverbal sounds are heard; recognizes tones and tunes but not words
Short-term memory decreases	Deterioration in verbal perception and selective improvement in all aspects of imaginal perception
Is unable to recognize winter and summer	Can easily select pairs of colors; is quick to evaluate unfinished drawings and identify defects
Visual disturbance	Loss of theoretical knowledge (schooling)
Is easygoing, sociable, cheerful, optimistic	Shapes and figures remain in harmony
	Loss of space orientation
	Loss of time orientation
	Is morose, pessimistic

*Note: The behaviors presented here are drawn from tests performed on sick people, so they will not necessarily apply to everyone. However, this practical information on breath-brain coordination will enable those now familiar with the right/left models of the holographic brain, or with various kinds of humanistic body work, to integrate the knowledge into their daily life and behavior.

his inner and outer world. Man is often distracted by a thought or an idea and begins to do whatever he feels like doing, without thinking about his present state of being. By watching the nostrils, and constantly keeping track of which side of the body is more active, he will develop the habit of coming back to a relaxed position. This practice will also enable him to decide if the activity should be done immediately or if he should wait until the nostril changes. He can also decide to change the nostril willfully.

CHAPTER 2

Swara Yoga and the Five Elements

S O FAR we have discussed the flow of the nasal
breath cycle, its relationship with nerves and nadis,
and its periodic alternation, which influences the
contralateral hemispheric dominance.

Swara Yoga also teaches us techniques to observe the
presence of the five elements in the body. Knowledge of
how these elements function will help us develop more
consciousness about the constituents of our feeling and
emotions. Yogic scriptures assert that true knowledge of
the Self is not possible without becoming *tattvatit* (going
beyond the elements). They also say one should become
tattvadarshi (an observer of the elements) because all
physiological and psychological changes arise from the
mutation of the *gunas* or qualities of nature and the
tattvas or elements. Swara Yoga provides a practical
means to observe these elements. Changes in body chemistry produce various psychological states. These

changes themselves have a periodic rhythm and a specific order. They are related to the five elements, which are the basis of all phenomenal existence. According to the ancient scriptures, the elements are the basis of all forms. The four elements—Earth, Water, Fire, and Air— were accepted by the Greeks and Egyptians; the Christians, Jews, and Muslims believed in these four elements. The fifth element, Akasha, was only known to the Indians. (The Chinese also believe in five elements, but they are Wood, Earth, Fire, Metal, and Water.)

In Yoga, Akasha holds the highest position because it is the source of the other four elements.

Before discussing how the elements and their attributes are revealed in the flow of the nasal breath, we will first describe them. Elements are agents of the primary inertia principle of consciousness. In evolution, three fields are created:

1. Mental-conscious field, created by *sattwa* (primary sentient principle)
2. Power field, created by *rajas* (primary energy principle; in this field, consciousness exists as frequencies and vibrations)
3. Material field, created by *tamas* (primary inert principle; in this field, consciousness exists in inert form)

Elements belong to the material field, which created antimatter and matter. They constitute a continuum of energy from the most subtle vibratory level to the most dense and gross vibrational level. At the grossest level of vibration, energy has substance (solidity), smell, taste, form, and touch (rough, smooth, even, uneven, etc.) and is inert, because it is a product of the inertia principle. This is known as the Earth element. In the Indian tradition, it is not the planet Earth that is known as the Earth element, but it is the Earth element that dominates the planet Earth. Smell is the characteristic of this element. For an example of the relationship of smell to the Earth element, we can look at the sandalwood tree in India: it can grow anywhere in the country, but the smell in the wood is absent because of the change of the soil. Where it grows naturally, the scent of sandalwood is strong. Similar discoveries were made with the seed of the Asian herb fenugreek. These seeds can be easily sprouted and grown outdoors or indoors, but the strong scent, which comes from the soil where the herb is naturally grown in India, is absent.

When excited into a higher frequency range, the Earth element loses its property of solidity. The substance becomes liquid and flowing, while still retaining the properties of form and touch. It penetrates through other things and becomes a binding material. Taste is the characteristic of this element. It is known that taste changes with a change in the water. The water element encompasses all substances in liquid form.

As the level of vibration increases, heat and light are generated by the accelerated motion. The property of liquidity vanishes and only the properties of form, touch, and sound remain. Energy at this level is called the Fire element. Form is the essential characteristic of the Fire element.

As the speed of the individual particles continues to accelerate, all form is lost, and heat and light are no longer produced. Now only the properties of touch and sound remain. Solidity, liquidity, and form all disappear. This is called the Air element. It is the prime mover.

Finally, when matter has lost all its tactile qualities, it reaches the most subtle layer of vibration. Sound is the characteristic that remains in the form of frequencies. This energy, in which matter exists in its etheric form, is known as the Akasha element.

In the evolution of the material field, which belongs to

the primary inertia principle, the energy exists as frequencies and slowly it materializes as Air, Fire, Water, and finally, Earth. Earth is the most dense, most cohesive form of this energy. Atoms are closely packed and structured with little freedom. In Water they are less densely assembled and the atoms are more dispersed, allowing a higher frequency range. In Fire the matter is less cohesive still, and in Air all semblance and cohesiveness vanishes. In Akasha, individual particles do not exist; only those vibrations that are beyond the material plane exist.

So far we have discussed only the material field, but as we mentioned earlier, in evolution the three fields operate simultaneously. The material field is permeated by the power field, which is created by the primary energy principle, prana or life force. This pranic energy operates in both the material and mental fields. Life force or pranic force transforms inorganic matter into living matter. This life force, which generates the power field, itself is pervaded by the mental-conscious field. The latter is generated by the primary sentient principle and provides the conscious power that selects appropriate materials to create an organism suitable for its manifestation. This transformation is brought about by a complicated process and the simple material substances become highly complex organisms.

In each living organism these three fields exist:

1. Material field, as physical body;
2. Power field, as life force or prana; and
3. Mental-conscious field, as individual consciousness.

These three fields are interwoven and everything exists at these three levels at the same time. For example, the material counterpart for each desire and feeling is present in the body's chemistry. Unless one understands this, it is difficult to overcome moods and high and low cycles; these are merely chemical changes related to the elements. Present-day scientists have gathered data to verify the influence of the Sun and the Moon on our moods. Paul Mirabile of the Institute of Living in Hartford, Connecticut, used a computerized database of four thousand psychiatric patients to confirm this ancient belief. The physical counterparts of the Sun and the Moon are the right and left nostrils, which operate through the action of the Pingala and Ida nadis. Their interplay on either side of the spinal column influences the chakras, the psychic centers that are directly connected with the five gross elements. Thus we see that elements play an important role in our behavior.

Specific centers in the subtle body function as seats for these elements (see Figures 6 and 7). The Tantric system, which has seven subtle centers or chakras, clearly acknowledges the lower five centers as the seat of five elements, i.e.,

1. Pelvic plexus—seat of the Earth element;
2. Hypogastric plexus—seat of the Water element;
3. Epigastric plexus—seat of the Fire element;
4. Cardiac plexus—seat of the Air element; and
5. Carotid plexus—seat of the Akasha element.

These centers are linked to the five sense organs and five work organs through a network of sympathetic and parasympathic nerves and subtle nadis.

With the operation of pranic force, these centers are activated in a natural rhythmic order. The five elements generate their respective frequencies, activating the sense organs and work organs related with them and thereby influencing the organism. By knowing the rhythmic order in which these centers are activated and the physiological impact they have, we can know the secrets

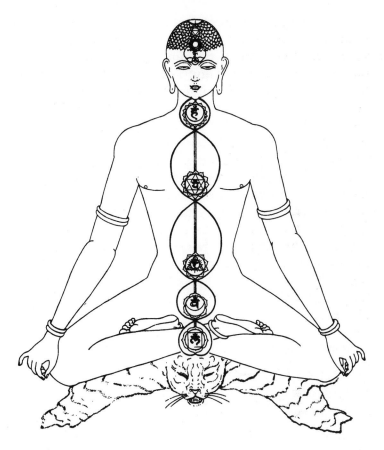

FIGURE 6.   The seven chakras seen inside a yogi meditating in the full Lotus posture.

of our feelings and emotions, and of our high and low cycles.

DURATION OF THE ELEMENTS

In the practice of Swara Yoga, the five elements come and go with each hourly cycle of the breath. The Air element is the starting point of the breath; each cycle of the nostrils begins with the Air element.

The order in which the elements prevail in the chakras or psychic centers of the body is as follows: first of all the Vayu (wind) element flows, followed by Agni (fire), Prithvi (earth), Varuna (water) and Akasha (sky) respectively (*Shiva Swarodaya,* v. 71). This order is different from the order in which the chakras are aligned along the central canal (as listed below, Earth to Akasha).

In one hour we breathe an average of 900 breaths (60 × 15 = 900). During these 900 breaths, each element dominates for a specific period of time:

> For 20 minutes (300 breaths) the Earth element dominates
>
> For 16 minutes (240 breaths) the Water element dominates
>
> For 12 minutes (180 breaths) the Fire element dominates
>
> For 8 minutes (120 breaths) the Air element dominates
>
> For 4 minutes (60 breaths) the Akasha element dominates

Of the sixty breaths of Akasha, Sushumna operates during the last ten. These ten breaths are the transitional moments before the other nostril takes over. Sushumna thus operates during each hour for a period of forty seconds. At sunrise and sunset it operates for a longer period of time, before the nostril of the day takes over. Meditation at sunrise and sunset, while the Sushumna breath flow is active, can bring electrochemical balance to the body. It can also extend the length of time the Sushumna is operative. Because the Sushumna breath is rooted in the central canal and thereby is connected with all the internal organs and chakras, it is best suited for meditation. This is one reason the seers of the Vedas, Upanishads and Tantras prescribed that worship be performed at dawn and dusk. None of the five elements work when the Sushumna operates, and all physical and mental desires are suspended. The mind becomes calm because no mental fluctuations exist at these times.

Mental fluctuations are prominent when either of the two nostrils is operative; they are more pronounced when the right nostril is operative. Until one begins to mark the flow of nasal breath and becomes aware of the relationship between the nostrils and the hemispheres, i.e., between breath and mind, one will not realize the importance of meditation and prolonging the period of Sushumna breath flow. By understanding the relationship between the breath and the elements and by constantly watching the proper synchronization of the nostrils, one can balance his or her own state of consciousness at will.

Living in Awareness

To live in constant awareness means that one should know what is happening inside, because the world outside is viewed by an individual according to his or her state of mind. When one is sad, the world outside appears to be quite different than when one is happy. Every individual is restricted by many invisible strings which comprise one's frame of reference. One's state of body chemistry provides the mood, feeling-tones, or emotional nuances with which to view the world outside. One has to develop witness-consciousness by watching one's actions, emotions, and thoughts objectively. In this regard, it is important to keep constant watch on one's nostrils and to understand that the world can only be perceived through the prism of one's own state of being at any given moment.

Watching the Elements

By watching the elements in each cycle of breath (see Figure 7), one can know very precisely the basis of thoughts and perception. This is done in eight steps.

1. Know the qualities of the elements.
2. Find the midpoint or juncture in the breath just before the nostrils switch over.
3. Determine the dominating nostril and know its nature.
4. Locate in which psychic center or chakra the breath is moving. We know that during each cycle of breath of sixty minutes (when the breath is operating through the right or left nostril) the Earth element, for example, dominates for twenty minutes. During this time period, one goes through the desires and activities, qualities and attributes connected with the Earth element. The seat of the Earth element is the pelvic plexus, so for those twenty minutes the location of breath would be the pelvic plexus. As stated earlier, the breath will begin with Air (eight minutes), Fire (twelve minutes) and then comes Earth (twenty minutes), Water (sixteen minutes) and finally Akasha (four minutes).
5. Watch the color of the element.
6. Measure the strength of exhalation, or prana.
7. Feel the dominant taste in the mouth, which is related to the element present.
8. Watch the direction the breath moves. Sometimes it

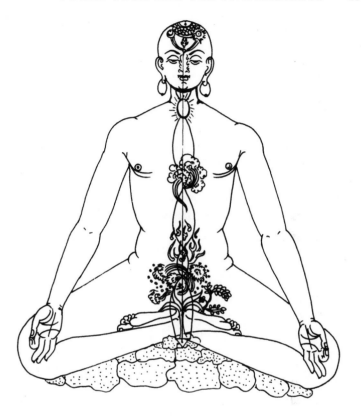

FIGURE 7. The elements seated within the chakras.

does not flow straight in and out of the nostril; for example, it can be angular and flow more towards the right or left side.

One should begin to determine which element is at play in the swara (dominant nostril) at the time of sunrise. Before the nostril of the day starts operating, the flow of air becomes bilaterally equal and Sushumna dominates. This joining period is known as *sandhi-kala* (*sandi*-joining; *kala*-period). This takes place half an hour before sunrise and is the starting point for the day).

Before starting to practice the science of watching the elements, one needs to know more about the nature of the elements.

NATURE OF THE ELEMENTS

Earth. The Earth element is situated in the *Muladhara* (pelvic plexis) and is connected with the central canal or Sushumna at its point of origin. The color of this element is yellow and its shape square. Smell is its predominant sense. The sense organ associated with the Earth element is the nose, and the work organ is the anus. The taste of the Earth element is sweet.

This element is best suited for stationary activities that require persistence. Worship done in the presence of this element brings *siddhis* or powers.

The Earth element extends from East to West and is beneficial during the day, for the preservation of life, for earning money, agriculture, victory and profit, and for enjoying the company of others. The Sun dominates when the Earth element is present in the right nostril breath. Knowledge of vegetation (trees, plants, etc.) becomes easy to grasp in the presence of this element.

Bones, flesh, skin, nadis, and body hairs belong to the Earth element and their growth is enhanced by the dominance of this element in the breath.

Each element is linked to a particular sound frequency called a seed sound or *bija* mantra. The seed sound of the Earth element is *LANG.* *

Diseases, such as jaundice, and mental ailments, such as phobias, are produced by a disturbance of the Earth element in the body.

---

*Although seed sounds are most often seen as ending in "m," according to the Tantrics the "ang" ending is more desirable; it vibrates in the Sahasrara and, as the sound moves through the nasal passage, it produces a special effect.

Water.   The Water element is situated in the *Swadhish-thana* (hypogastric plexus). The color of this element is white and its shape is like a crescent moon or half moon. Taste is its predominant sense. Its sense organ is the tongue and its work organ the genitals. The taste is saline.

The Water element is best suited for movement and activity. Worship in the presence of this element, as with the Earth element, brings power.

The presence of the Water element is beneficial at night and its direction is West. The Moon dominates when this element is present in the left nostril breath. Knowledge of auspicious works becomes easy to grasp.

Semen, blood, fat, urine, mucus, saliva, and lymphatic fluids belong to the water element.

The seed sound of this element is *VANG*.

Emotional disorders are related to a disturbance in the water element in the body.

Fire.   The Fire element is situated in the *Manipura* (epigastric plexus; solar plexus). The color of this element is red and its shape is triangular. Sight is the predominant sense of this element. Eyes are the sense organs and feet and legs are the work organs. The taste is bitter.

The Fire element is best suited to obtaining knowledge of a mental nature and performing destructive actions. It produces more energy when the breath is flowing through the right nostril; it brings success in all good and bad work. Mars dominates in the presence of the Fire element when the breath is flowing through the right nostril. The direction connected with this element is South.

Hunger, thirst, sleep, lethargy, and radiance (*ojas*) are related to the Fire element.

The seed sound of this element is *RANG*.

Disorders like anger, stomach ailments, and swelling in

the body are caused by disturbance in the Fire element. The presence of this element facilitates the process of awakening the Kundalini. Meditation on this element gives a tremendous appetite, tolerance for sunshine or fire, and removes indigestion and other stomach disorders.

Air. The Air element is situated in the *Anahata* (cardiac plexus; heart). The color of this element is smoky green and its shape as seen on a mirror or a piece of glass is oval. Touch is the predominant sense of this element. Skin is the sense organ and hands the work organ. The taste is sour.

Its presence produces restlessness. Actvities that require movement can be successfully done in the presence of the Air element.

Rahu (the north node of the Moon or the Dragon's Head) dominates when the Air element is present and dominant in the right nostril. The direction connected with the air element is North.

The seed sound is *YANG*.

Disorders created by the aggravation of the humor of Air include dryness of skin, skin diseases, and diseases of the nervous system. Heart diseases, high blood pressure, stress, loneliness, pessimism, and depression are caused by wind disorders as well.

Akasha.   The Akasha element is situated in the *Vishuddha* (carotid plexus; throat). The color of this element is smoky purple and its shape, as seen on a mirror or piece of glass, is oval. Hearing is the predominant sense. Ears are its sense organs and the mouth (vocal cords) are the work organ of this element. Bitter is its taste.

The Akasha element is not suitable for worldly activities because it spoils everything done in its dominance. The scriptures say the Akasha element makes everything infructuous—it gives inauspicious results, causes loss and death. However yoga *sadhana* (practice of yoga and meditation) can be done in its presence.

The seed sound of Akasha is *HANG.*

This element is situated in the middle of all directions.

Love, enmity, shyness, fear, and attachment are five qualities of Akasha. Jupiter dominates when the element is dominant in the left nostril. Meditation on Akasha with the repetition of its *bija* mantra brings knowledge of past, present, and future and bestows the eight well-known *siddhis:*

1. *Anima*—atomicity
2. *Laghima*—lightness
3. *Mahima*—mightiness
4. *Ishvata*—power over others
5. *Vasitva*—attraction over others
6. *Prakam*—assuming a desired form
7. *Bhukti*—power to enjoy
8. *Prapti*—attainments of all kinds

Techniques for Detecting the Elements

Now that we have examined the nature of the five elements, we may begin "watching" them.

1. The exact location of the passing air in the nostril can reveal which of the five elements is active in the system at a particular time.
2. The shape formed by the vapor deposit on a piece of glass following an exhale can reveal the dominant element.

3. By performing *Yoni Mudra* (see page 48), the color of the element is seen.

4. By measuring the force of the exhaled breath, the length of the breath and thus the element can be ascertained.

LOCATION OF BREATH IN THE NOSTRILS

If the exhaled air passes through a particular spot in the nostril, or moves in a specific manner, it indicates the dominance of one element:

- Center of the nostril—Earth element
- Lower part of the nostril—Water element
- Top of the nostril—Fire element
- Obliquely through the side of the nostril—Air element
- Rotating in the nostril—Akasha element*

SHAPE OF THE ELEMENT

To find out which element is present at a given moment, one should place the top of the nose on a piece of glass, a windowpane, or a mirror and exhale forcefully several times. The vapors will soon start to evaporate. If one watches carefully, however, one can see a figure emerging from the haze (see Figure 8).

---

*"If the swara flows in the upward direction, it indicates death; its downward flow gives tranquility. When it flows in an oblique manner, the Swara yogi can do the Tantric act of *uchchatan* (act of repelling others), the Tantric karma of *stambhan* (paralyzing others), and obstructive acts not socially desirable. These Tantric acts cannot be done successfully in the presence of the Akasha element; a Swara yogi should avoid any Tantric karma in its presence."

Shiva Swaradaya, v. 159

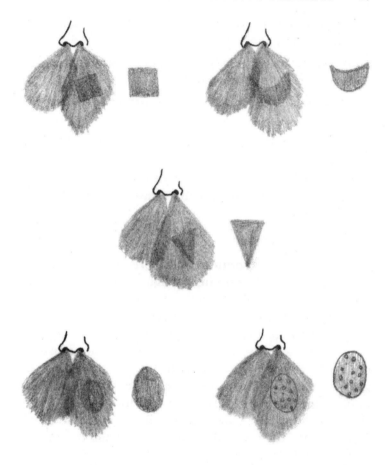

FIGURE 8.   Five patterns formed by exhalation of breath. A square form indicated the presence of the Earth element, which dominates for twenty minutes. A crescent shape indicates the presence of the Water element, which dominates for sixteen minutes. A triangular form indicates the presence of the Fire element, which dominates for twelve minutes. An oval form indicates the presence of the Air element, which dominates for eight minutes. An oval shape with small droplets of water indicates the Akasha element, which dominates for four minutes.

- A square shape indicates the presence of the Earth element.

- A crescent shape (half moon shape) indicates the presence of the Water element.

- A triangular shape indicates the presence of the Fire element.

- An oval shape indicates the presence of the Air element.

- An oval shape formed by tiny drops of water or spots indicates the presence of the Akasha element.

COLOR OF THE ELEMENT

Another method of confirming the presence of a particular element is by assuming a yogic posture called the *Yoni Mudra*. Place the right and left thumbs on the openings of the ears and press them shut; with the middle fingers of each hand, one should close the two nostrils. Then place the two index fingers on closed eyelids and apply a little pressure. With the two remaining fingers—the third finger and the little finger of both hands—one should tightly close the lips.

Before doing the Yoni Mudra, one should take a full, deep breath. After a while, colors will begin to emerge. The process can be facilitated by increasing the pressure on the eyelids.

- The presence of yellow denotes the Earth element.

- The presence of white indicates the Water element.

- Presence of red indicates the Fire element.

- Presence of smoky green or black indicates the Air element.

- When one sees small spots of many colors, the presence of Akasha is indicated.

LENGTH OF THE BREATH

The length of the breath also provides a clue to determining which element is present in the nasal breath at any given time. To measure the length of the exhaled breath one should place a piece of fine cotton on a small piece of cardboard. Then bring the cardboard with the fine cotton on it towards the operating nostril and exhale. The exhaled breath will begin to act on the cotton at a distance, and that movement will gradually become visible. The point where the cotton ball starts moving with the force of the exhaled breath is the strength of the breath; it is also known as the length of the breath.

The technique described above is very ancient. The point where the cotton ball starts showing its effect of the exhaled breath is then measured by fingers, because the nostrils and fingers of the same person will have a proportionate relationship. This measurement in the scriptures is called finger widths. (Perhaps a quicker and more accurate method of measuring the length and strength of the breath could be designed.)

- The strength of the Earth element is 12 finger widths.
- The strength of the Water element is 16 finger widths.
- The strength of the Fire element is 4 finger widths.
- The strength of the Air element is 8 finger widths.
- The strength of the Akash element is 20 finger widths.

The taste of the elements (see chart, page 52) can also be discerned in the mouth. This provides one more key to determining the presence of an element. The taste should be experienced at the time one performs the *Yoni Mudra** and sees the color of the element.

*Note: Smokers should refrain from smoking at least a half hour before doing the Yoni Mudra and should rinse their mouth thoroughly, otherwise the taste will not be recognized.

Change in Length of the Breath and Its Influence

In Chapter 1, we discussed the normal rhythm of breathing and mentioned that by reducing the number of breaths one's life span can be prolonged. Now we will discuss not the quantity of breaths, but the size or length of the breath. One can achieve all kinds of states and powers if the breath length is reduced. The normal breath length is ten finger widths for an inhale (*pooraka*) and twelve finger widths for an exhale (*rechaka*).

The length of the breath changes, depending upon the physical act one is engaged in:

> In singing, the length increases to 16 finger widths.
>
> In eating and vomiting, the length increases to 18 finger widths.
>
> In walking, the length increases to 24 finger widths.
>
> In running, the length increases to 30 finger widths.
>
> At the time of sexual intercourse, the length is 65 finger widths.

The techniques to reduce the length of the breath can only be learned from a Guru in person. No amount of study from books can provide this knowledge. Some pure souls obtain this knowledge due to their past karmas and the grace of the Guru. A teacher who has mastered these techniques and can practice them has the power to disappear and become invisible at will. He will be visible only if the student is favored by luck and has divine support. So it is best to simply practice Swara Yoga and

Table 4. Benefits of Reducing Breath Length

REDUCTION OF FINGER WIDTHS	
From 12 to 11	Desirelessness and stabilization of prana
From 12 to 10	Tranquility, calmness, bliss
From 12 to 9	Ability to compose poetry
From 12 to 8	Perfection in language and power of speech
From 12 to 7	See far-off places; clairvoyance
From 12 to 6	Power to fly in air and sky
From 12 to 5	Tremendous speed of movement
From 12 to 4	Siddhis: *anima* (atomicity), *laghima* (lightness), *mahima* (mightiness)
From 12 to 3	Divine treasures
From 12 to 2	Siddhi known as *prakam* (power to assume any form at will)
From 12 to 1	Siddhi known as *sarvakam* (power to appear, disappear, and fulfill all desires)

to try to reduce the number of breaths per minute. This practice itself can provide good luck and draw divine support.

The chart of elements (see page 52) will facilitate a broad understanding of the elements.

The Chart of Elements at a Glance

NAME OF THE ELEMENT	LOCATION IN THE BODY (CHAKRA)	SHAPE	GUNA OR CHARACTER-ISTIC	COLOR	TASTE	ATTRIBUTE
Earth	Muladhara (Pelvic Plexus) 1st Chakra	Square □	Smell	Yellow	Sweet	Greed
Water	Swadhishthana (Hypogastric Plexus) 2nd Chakra	Half Moon ☽	Taste	White	Saline/ Astringent	Attachment
Fire	Manipura (Epigastric Plexus) 3rd Chakra	Triangle △	Form	Red	Bitter Hot Pungent	Anger
Air	Anahata (Cardiac Plexus) 4th Chakra	Oval or Round ○	Touch	Smoky Green	Sour	Sex
Akasha	Vishuddha (Carotid Plexus) 5th Chakra	Oval with Dots	Sound	Smoky Violet	Bitter Like Quinine	Egotism

NOTE: The duration of elements is calculated on a one-hour cycle of breath through one of the nostrils as stated in *Shiva Swarodaya* and *Gyana Swarodaya*, the scriptures of Swara Yoga. Experiments conducted by neurobiologists suggest that the duration in United States is between two to three hours. Neurophysiologists conducted research on circadian rhythms and discovered a 2-hour cycle of nares (in adults). The difference may be due to the difference of climate between India and the United States.

NATURE	DESIRE	ACTIVITY	BIJA SEED SOUND	FLOW OF BREATH IN NOSTRILS	LENGTH OF BREATH	DURATION
Stable	To Survive	Collecting, Saving	Lang ॐ लं	Center of the Nostrils	Twelve Finger Widths	Twenty Minutes
Cool Unstable	Meeting People	Peaceful Auspicious	Vang ॐ वं	Lower Part of the Nostrils	Sixteen Finger Widths	Sixteen Minutes
Hot-Headed	Achieve-ment	Hard Labor	Rang ॐ रं	Upper Area of the Nostrils	Four Finger Widths	Twelve Minutes
Restless	Activity Movement	Temporary Jobs	Yang ॐ यं	Sideways Oblique	Eight Finger Widths	Eight Minutes
Void	To Be Alone	Thoughts and Ideas	Hang ॐ हं	Circular Rotating	Twenty Finger Widths	Four Minutes

The Earth element gives considerable success in stable work; the Water element gives immediate gains in unstable work; the Fire element gives middling results; the Air element produces loss; and the Akasha element makes things unsuccessful.

Earth nourishes the physical body, the muscles, bones, and hairs. Water nourishes bodily fluids, i.e., blood, lymph, etc. Fire nourishes the digestive fire and ojas (the radiance). Air nourishes prana, the circulatory system, endocrine glands, nerves, and skin. Akasha nourishes the ears, semen, and brain.

CHAPTER 3

Healing and Other Applications of Swara Yoga

S WARA YOGA introduces a technology that makes any and every practitioner able to get away from an unwanted emotional state. In the words of Dr. Shannahoff-Khalsa: "If you want to alter an unwanted state, just breathe through the more congested nostril." According to Dr. Khalsa, the knowledge of this ancient technology enables anyone to correct his or her own mental and physical imbalances.* In this way Swara Yoga can be of great help in healing oneself.

With Swara Yoga one can not only help ones own emotional state and heal the physical body, but can create favorable conditions for one's life by changing the environment and improving one's living conditions. In addition, one can foretell death, determine the sex of a child not yet conceived, and heal others around us.

*Brain Mind Bulletin, Vol. 8, No. 3, Jan. 3, 1983.

Healing Oneself

Our moods sometimes create electrochemical disturbance in the body. When we remain in one state of mind for an extended period of time, the natural rhythmic cycle of the elements is disturbed. Because the elements form the physical reality of our psychological responses, one particular chemical environment can dominate within our body.

By knowledge and practice of Swara Yoga, we can develop a habit of watching ourselves and the operating nostril. We can notice when one nostril is dominant for longer than its normal cycle duration and change it.

By changing the operating nostril, we change the active side of the body, its glandular secretions, and reestablish a chemical balance. Swara Yoga advises changing the operating nostril at the first sign of any physical or mental disturbance. This prevents worsening of the symptoms and promotes rapid recovery.

If one is not fully alert at the time one receives the first signal from within the body, the operating nostril should be changed as soon as one remembers or feels an unwanted state.

Sometimes ailments are created by exposure to extreme cold or heat, infections, and viruses. These conditions can also be cured by a change of the nostrils.

Fever: When the body temperature increases, one should plug the operating nostril with a cotton ball and keep it plugged until the body comes back to normal. Usually the right nostril becomes dominant in fever, but in fever caused by catching cold it can be the reverse. So one should follow the rule of plugging the operating nostril.

Indigestion: Chronic indigestion can be cured by cultivating a habit of eating only when the right nostril is working and by drinking lukewarm water when indigestion is felt. Drinking lukewarm water only when the left nostril is working helps and cures indigestion; adding the juice of one lemon provides an additional benefit.

Those patients with chronic indigestion should cultivate a habit of lying on the left side fifteen to twenty minutes before each meal, and for the same period of time after eating.

Taking a half teaspoon of oregano seeds, with a pinch of salt in warm water, cures indigestion that is not chronic.

To lie on the left side before food for a period of fifteen to twenty minutes is healthy for all human beings. This practice should be followed by a nice, leisurely walk.

The rules for good digestion are as follows:

1. After eating, lie on the back and breathe eight rounds (one inhale and one exhale per round), then;

2. Change to the right side and breathe sixteen rounds through the left nostril;

3. Change to the left side and breathe thirty-two rounds through the right nostril. Then, if you can relax longer, remain on your left side and continue breathing from the right nostril. Listen to joyful and uplifting music. Music that creates a meditative mood or state after eating will disturb the body chemistry and create indigestion.

Those who are able to sit in the Lotus posture should do so. If one has had a bowel movement but has not eaten anything, this exercise can be done at any time of the day. In this posture, one can gaze at the navel steadily for about ten to fifteen minutes. This practice should not be done unless one has had a bowel movement. Meditation on the navel with silent repetition of the bija mantra of the Manipura chakra—*RANG*—helps. This is also the bija of the Fire element, and its repetition will increase digestive fire and help to cure all stomach ailments.

By cultivating a habit of defecating before sunrise and only when the right nostril is working, one can cure numerous physical and mental problems created by toxins in the intestines.

Constipation: Eating and defecating only when the right nostril is open, and lying down on the left side before and after eating, helps constipation. One should also drink a moderate amount of liquids when the left nostril is working.

Breathing exercises, or pranayama, and walking in the morning or after dinner are also helpful. Avoid coffee or tea after meals; drink prune juice and lukewarm water; use wheat germ in cereals; eat green leafy vegetables, squash, zucchini, and coconut powder. Milk heated and sweetened with dates taken before going to bed is also good. Eating figs with breakfast and prunes after meals also provides additional help. Listening to the sound of drumming can aid in the cure of constipation.

Stress: Stress created by hard work and physical labor can be cured by lying on the right side and breathing through the left nostril for twenty-five to thirty minutes.

Listening to music that creates a meditative mood can also alleviate stress. Harp, zither, and other string instruments are especially effective. A gentle foot massage and combing the hair with the fingers or a wooden comb can provide relief. Before lying down on the right side, one's feet, hands, and face should be washed and the mouth rinsed. Cool the eyes with moderately cold water after rinsing the mouth to provide a fresh feeling and aid the healing process.

To relieve stress caused by physical exertion, one

should drink a glass of warm milk sweetened by dates after relaxing on the right side for twenty-five to thirty minutes; a pinch of saffron added to the milk brings happiness.

Joint pain: For recurring pain in the joints, changing the nostril is always helpful. The following treatment is prescribed as well.

Lie on the back for five minutes after the morning cleansing (bowel movement) and then change to the right side and breathe through the left nostril for fifteen to twenty minutes. Follow this routine for a two-week period. A massage of the painful area with Mahanarayana Oil and a drink of fenugreek tea* is also helpful.

Neck pain: First change the operating nostril. Then hold the shoulders with both hands and move them in a circular direction, as if you were rowing a boat.

When the pain in the neck is recurrent:

1. Apply dry heat to the neck area
2. Massage with a soothing massage oil
3. Lie in the Corpse Posture while the left nostril is operating

Back pain: After changing the nostril, one should follow the procedure that follows:

---

*Note: To make fenugreek tea, have the following ingredients ready: fenugreek seeds, milk, fresh ginger, and black peppercorns. Boil 2 cups of water with 2½ grams of fresh ginger (do not use dry or powdered ginger) and ½ teaspoon of fenugreek seeds for fifteen minutes. When half the water boils away, add half a cup of milk and 7 black peppercorns; let the mixture come just to the boiling point. Remove from the heat, strain, and add raw sugar to taste. (Do not use honey as a sweetener in the tea; honey should not be heated or used in hot milk or tea.) Drink the tea while it is warm. Make sure that your left nostril is working when you ingest the tea.

1. Take a small amount of beeswax, warm it slightly, and mold it into small balls, about the combined size of three peas. Take internally with warm milk that has been boiled with ½ teaspoon of fenugreek seeds. Swallowing one ball each day for forty days cures most chronic backaches except those caused by physical injury or nervous disorders. Try this method for ten days and watch for the effect on the pain. If the problem disappears, one can stop the treatment. If the problem is not cured, one should continue for ten more days, stop for a week, and observe the painful area. This way one can determine how much medicine is needed. Forty days is the maximum period of time this treatment should be used.

2. One should avoid the use of the following foods: rice; dry beans; yogurt; eggplant; cauliflower; canned foods; foods that have been cooked more than eight hours before they are eaten; fried foods; hot spices; and excessive use of salt.

Headache: After changing the nostril, one should follow the procedure listed below:

1. Plug the operating nostril with a cotton ball until the headache pain is gone. This is the first thing one should do under ordinary circumstances. It does not help when the headache comes during the period of menstruation, or is caused by a disturbance in the body gases.

2. Find the carotid arteries, located in the neck grooves to each side of the Adam's apple. Press these arteries with the thumbs.

3. Induce sneezing by snuff.

4. While lying on the back in a corpse pose, tie a piece of cloth around each bicep muscle (middle of the upper

arm), and breathe through the left nostril. This technique cures a headache within ten to fifteen minutes.

Asthma: When asthmatic symptoms are first noticed, the patient should determine the operating nostril and plug it until the symptoms disappear. Following this remedy for one month at the first sign of the symptoms helps cure asthma permanently.

Meditation on the Anahata chakra, or heart center, with silent repetition of the bija sound associated with the fourth chakra—*YANG*—is beneficial.

Wet dreams: Sitting in *Siddhasana* after the morning bowel movement for half an hour daily while concentrating on the navel cures wet dreams. This practice must be followed every day for six months. Eating cereal cooked with water chestnut flour (*halwa*)* for breakfast will help.

Healing Others

Healing or helping a sick person can be done with or without the administration of medicine. In either case, the healer can follow the advice of the Swara yogis: to develop psychic powers through willpower and to give the healing or medication while attentive to his or her own nostril dominance. The healer should follow the procedure listed below:

1. Observe the patient's operating nostril, and help the patient to change the breath flow.

---

*To make halwa, place half a cup of water chestnut flour dry in a frying pan. Add a little ghee or butter and roast until the flour becomes brown. Add a cup of water and stir until it becomes a thick paste. Add 2 to 3 tablespoons of raw sugar, 2 teaspoons ghee or butter, 1 green cardamom, powdered, and 7 black peppercorns, ground and powdered. Heat three minutes and serve.

2. By using the power of one's own operating nostril at specific times. For example, the healer should give medication with the right hand, when his or her own right nostril is working and with the left hand, when his or her own left nostril is working. The healer should also exhale from his or her operating nostril onto the medication before giving it to the patient. The patient should be kept on the side of the healer's operating nostril. The healer then breathes out from his or her operating nostril into the non-operating nostril of the patient.

Creating Favorable Conditions

The operating nostril can be very effectively used to create favorable conditions. Whenever it is desirable to influence another person, one should first find out which nostril is operative. Then one should approach the person on that side. For example, if one's right nostril is operating, the person to be influenced should be positioned either to one's right, below, or behind. If one's left nostril is operating, the person to be influenced should be to one's left, above, or in front.

When applying for employment, one should mark his or her operating nostril. In addition, one should initiate or step out with the foot that corresponds to the operating nostril. That is, the right foot when the right nostril is working and vice versa.

Another important thing to remember at this time is that the right nostril is solar and is connected with odd numbers, and the lunar or left nostril is connected with even numbers. When the right nostril is working, one should proceed with the right foot and take the first three steps with the right foot. When the left nostril is working, one should proceed with the left foot, and take the first four steps with the left foot.

Upon reaching one's destination, check the nostrils again and step into the building or room leading with the foot that corresponds to the operating nostril.

If one has to meet someone important, one should follow the instructions given above and position the person on the side of one's operating nostril. Such a meeting will be fruitful.

In addition, one should attempt to mark which element is present in the operative nostril at the time one is seeking to schedule an interview and make note of it. If Earth or Water elements are present, the position will certainly be secured. In the presence of the Fire element, the position will be secured with some difficulties. In the presence of the Air or Akasha element, one should avoid scheduling the interview and call at another time.

In addition to applying for employment, attending meetings, etc., the practices given above yield fruitful results in other life situations as well.

Improving One's Living Conditions

In addition to following the above procedures, when it is desirable to increase one's prosperity and secure better living conditions, one should:

1. Get up each day at least half an hour before sunrise.
2. Before getting out of bed, or seeing or talking with anyone, one should complete the following practice:
   - Find out which nostril is dominant.
   - Kiss the palm of the hand that corresponds with the operative nostril (right palm when the right nostril is working, and vice versa).
   - With the same hand, rub the face, head, neck, chest, thighs, and feet.

- Step out of bed, placing the foot that corresponds with the operating nostril on the ground or floor first.
- Proceed with morning cleansing (bowel movement, cleaning of mouth, etc.).

This daily practice will improve the conditions of one's life. One achieves better living situations and prosperity and is considered by others to be a lucky person.

Foretelling Death

Life and death are two sides of the manifested Consciousness. They are the eternal pair of opposites that play continuously with each other. To some people, death can be a horrible thought, but to those who know the mysteries, death is just a change of form. Although Consciousness needs a physical vehicle to operate in, its nature is the never-changing, eternal reality—the absolute Truth; it does not die with the body. Death is in fact a point of relief. To those who see death as a pleasant change, it might be interesting to know about the moment of death, or how far they are from their own point of release. The following guidelines on nasal breath flow will be useful in determining length of life.

1. If the right nostril operates for 24 hours in a row, the person will live for three more years and then leave his or her body, or die.
2. If the right nostril operates for 48 hours in a row, the person will live for two more years and then leave the body.
3. If the right nostril operates for 120 hours (five days and five nights) in a row, then the person lives for one more year.

4. If the right nostril operates for 15 days in a row, or if the right nostril operates during the day and the left nostril operates at night for one month in a row, the person survives for six months.

5. If the right nostril operates for 20 days in a row, the person survives for three more months.

6. If the right nostril operates for 30 days in a row, the person survives for only two days.

7. If the left nostril operates all the time for more than two weeks, and the right nostril does not flow at all, one month of life is left.

8. If no nasal breath whatsoever is operating and a person starts breathing through the mouth, he or she will die within 96 minutes.

9. If the Sushumna operates for two hours in a row, one dies instantaneously.

10. If a person cannot see his or her own nose or tongue, he or she dies within three days.

11. If the heart region, feet, and scalp get dry after bathing, without using a towel, then the person dies within three months.

12. If a thin person suddenly becomes fat, or a fat person thin; if a weak person becomes strong, or a strong person weak; if a black person becomes fair, or a fair person dark; if a religious person becomes irreligious, etc., he or she dies within eight months.

13. If the breath of a person flows day and night through one nostril alone, that person should understand that only three years of life are left.

The following experiments offer other ways to determine length of life:

1. Place your right fist on your forehead, in straight

alignment with the nose. Stare at the lower arm. You will notice that, after a few minutes, the arm will appear to be very thin.

When the wrist begins to appear very thin and starts disappearing, and the arm divides in your vision into two pieces—completely disconnected from the wrist—it indicates that only six months are left.

2. One should take a pot full of water and, while facing East, look at the reflection of the Sun. If the reflection does not form a perfect circle, but is cut in any of the four dirctions—East, West, North, or South—the length of life should be understood as follows:

> Reflection cut in an easterly direction: life span is 1 month
>
> Reflection cut in a westerly direction: life span is 3 months
>
> Reflection cut in a northerly direction: life span is 2 months
>
> Reflection cut in a southerly direction: life span is 6 months
>
> If a hole appears in the center of the Sun's reflection, a life span of ten days remains.
>
> If the entire Sun disc seems to be rotating, the person will die on the same day.

3. One who cannot see the Sun, the Moon, fire, and their rays, will live only for eleven months.

4. A person who develops pain in the palm of the hand or the root of the tongue, whose blood becomes dark, and who feels no pain, even when pinched, dies within seven months.

5. If the wind, urine, and stools all come out at the same time, a person will survive for ten more days. (In a healthy person, the urine should precede the stools.)

6. If one does not see a light spot within the eyes when
   the inner corners are lightly pressed, the person will
   survive for ten more days.

Determining the Sex of a Child

The first thing to remember when attempting to affect
the sex of one's offspring is that a man is more male
when his right nostril is working, and a woman is more
female when her left nostril is operating.

To have sexual intercourse when the man breathes
through his right nostril and the woman through her left
is ideal.

Whenever a couple desires a son, they should only
engage in sex after the woman has menstruated. The
man's right nostril and the woman's left nostril should be
operating during intercourse. The element present in the
man should be either Earth or Water, or a combination of
both these elements. As well, it should be either the
eighth, tenth, twelfth, fourteenth, or sixteenth night after the purification brought by the menstrual cycle. The
latter period is better for purposes of fertilization. The
period just following the menstrual cycle is not good for
producing offspring:

> Fertilization on the fourth night following the
> menstrual cycle produces a son who is short-
> lived and poor.
>
> On the sixth night, it produces a son with an
> average life span.
>
> On the eighth night, it produces a son who lives
> a prosperous and successful life.
>
> On the tenth night, it produces a son who is
> smart, wise, and practical.

On the twelfth night, a son with virtues.

On the fourteenth night, a son who has superior qualities, beauty, wealth, and a name.

And on the sixteenth night, the son will have all virtues; he will be handsome, wealthy, prosperous, internationally famous, and will give comfort to others.

If the conception takes place when the right nostril of the man and the left nostril of the woman is working, and the Earth element is dominant, the son will be famous, virtuous, prosperous, and handsome.

If conceived in the Water element, the son will be comfort-giving, obedient, virtuous, and wealthy. He will never become poor.

If conceived in the Fire element, the son's life will be short; there are even chances of an abortion.

If conceived in the Air element, the progeny will bring pain and problems.

If conception takes place in the Akasha element, this will lead to an abortion, as is the case when sexual intercourse takes place during Sushumna.

The Swara Yoga scriptures, *Shiva Swarodaya* and *Gyana Swarodaya*, do not mention the subject of producing a daughter. However, a special article on the spiritual practices of Swara Yoga published in a noted Indian journal* does give the following information on this subject.

To produce a daughter, the couple should engage in sexual intercourse when the man's left nostril and the woman's right nostril are operating, and the Water element is reigning.

Kaylan, printed in Sadhna Ank, published in 1942 by Geeta Press, Gorakhpur, U.P., India.

Conception on the fifth night produces a daughter who gives birth to sons.

Conception on the seventh night produces a daughter who will be sterile.

Conception on the ninth night produces a daughter who will be prosperous, beautiful, and virtuous.

Conception on the eleventh night produces a daughter who will have a bad character.

Conception on the thirteenth night produces a daughter who will marry in some other caste and produce a hybrid generation.

Conception on the fifteenth night produces a daughter who will be beautiful, fortunate, prosperous, and will be married to a king or a wealthy man with noble qualities.

Sexual intercourse with a sterile woman, when the Fire element and either the right nostril or the Sushumna is operating in a man (whether during the day or night), should make the sterile woman become pregnant.

If conception takes place on the odd days after menstruation, when the Earth, Water, or Fire elements are present, and when the right nostril is dominant in a man (whether during the day or night), and the left nostril is flowing in a woman, the sterile woman should bear a child.

CHAPTER 4

Overview of Swara Yoga

S WARA YOGA is a precise, holistic branch of knowledge and the most practical science discovered by Tantra. It is the yoga of right living—of living in awareness and living like a wise person.

The nose can be seen as the main switch of the cerebral hemispheres. It can stimulate electromagnetic activity on one side of the body; it can switch the hemispheric activity on and off at will.

The nasal cycle and elements, combined together, organize the psychophysical theatre of life (*leela*). The chakras or psychic centers are the playground of the elements: with the rise of breath in one nostril, the game starts with the Air element and ends with the Akasha. The main connection between prana and the chakras is established by the three main nadis—Ida, Pingala, and Sushumna. These nadis are directly influenced by the swara (the breath operating through either of the nostrils) that is dominant, because breathing itself is a neuro-motor action and cannot be performed without the com-bined operation of nerves and nadis. The nadis connect the nostrils with the chakras and with the elements. As discussed earlier, the presence of different elements brings a change of taste to the mouth, indicating a change in the body chemistry. Energy flows through the chakras, which is seen as a change in the elements. It flows with a special rhythm (see sequence given on page 38). In nor-mal human beings the duration of Sushumna is too short, only ten breaths, but when one starts doing Swara Yoga this time period can be extended and energy can flow in the upper chakras for a longer time.

The emergence and dissolution of the elements influ-ences the three main body humors, known in Ayurveda as the three *doshas*:

1. Wind (*vayu*)—produced by the Air element
2. Bile (*pitta*)—produced by the Fire element
3. Mucus (*kapha*)—produced by the combination of Earth and Water elements

These humors create temperament. The chemical na-ture of man is established in the body chemistry at the time the ovum is fertilized. The body pattern of each individual depends on the condition of the mother. Ac-cording to Ayurveda, there are five factors that deter-mine the body chemistry of the unborn child:

1. Body chemistry of the father at the time of inter-course, which determines the chemical nature of the sperm.
2. Body chemistry of the mother, which determines the genetic chemicals in the ovum.
3. Food taken by the father and mother in the thirty-six hours prior to intercourse.

4. Emotional response of the mother, from the time of intercourse to the point of actual conception.
5. The general condition of the womb itself, the mucus lining the internal organs, and the chemical substance that lines the inner walls of the passage leading to the womb.

It is through these body humors that the human organism accepts the environmental changes and receives energy from food. The whole human organism is governed by wind, bile and mucus, which are the physiological counterparts to the elements.

Breath is the connecting link between the three humors, the five elements, the seven chakras, and the electrochemical changes that take place in the two hemispheres of the brain.

Meditation and Visualization Practices

Swara Yoga does not look at the body as comprised of individual parts or units; it fuses all the ingredients into one whole, and it gives practical methods for enhancing mental and physical well-being, along with spiritual evolution. All yogas and disciplines are incomplete without the knowledge of the swaras. Swara Yoga teaches us to take action when the right environment, inside and outside, is present. It teaches us to conserve energy and make the best use of our energy by keeping constant awareness of the working principle in our body, the breath.

Swara Yoga encompasses much more, including knowledge of past, present, and future, but to cover this information would require a separate book. Another title on *Breath Astrology* is forthcoming from this author and will be printed at a later time. If practitioners of Swara Yoga would verify the information contained in this book by direct experience, they would have a better life and an improved awareness.

The sound "So Ham," the natural sound of the inhalation and exhalation of breath, constantly points towards the oneness of all existing Consciousness. It serves to continually remind each one of us that we are that same energy which pervades the entire world of names and forms. With each inhalation, the sound "So" is made, and with each exhalation, the sound "Ham" is made; combined the sound becomes *So Ham* which, in Sanskrit, means "I am That" (So = that; aham = I am). With each breath this sound is constantly repeated without any conscious effort, without the help of vocal cords. As one listens to the sound of the breath, So Ham quiets the mind and allows the individual consciousness to transcend the body/mind limitations. By meditating on the sound So Ham one becomes enlightened and gets the knowledge of the past, present, and future. Swara Yoga prescribes ongoing meditation on So Ham, the natural sound of breath.

Other specific practices of Swara Yoga consist of: (1) synchronizing all mental and physical activities with the operating nostril; (2) following the Yamas or disciplines, such as non-violence, truth, honesty, sexual continence, forbearance, fortitude, kindness, straightforwardness, moderation in diet, and purity; (3) following the Niyamas or observances, which include austerity, contentment, and charity; and (4) visualizing and meditating on the chakras.

We have already discussed at length the first point mentioned above. The benefits to be derived from points two and three, the foundation of all yogas, are self-evident. Now we will discuss briefly the practice of visualizing and meditating on the chakras—the playground of the elements.* Visualization can be best accomplished

---

*Harish Johari, *Chakras* (Rochester, Vermont: Destiny Books, 1987).

when the breath changes from one nostril to the other. The element also changes at this time, spontaneously activating its corresponding chakra.

Since each hourly cycle of the nostrils begins with the Air element, this element becomes the starting point for the practice. While focusing attention on the Heart chakra (Anahata), which corresponds to the Air element, one must continuously repeat the bija-mantra of this element—YANG (see chart on page 53). The bija-mantra of an element and the seed sound of its corresponding chakra are the same. The meditation should begin with the aspirant visualizing each of the chakra petals. Each visualization should be followed by a repetition of the sound for that petal. Next the aspirant should meditate on the yantra of the Anahata chakra—the smoky-green six pointed star. This visualization is followed by meditation on the animal associated with the chakra, the deer (black antelope); the animal should be perceived as the carrier of the bija sound, in this case YANG. The aspirant continues by first focusing on the beautiful Kundalini Shakti, seated in lotus posture within a triangle, and then on Shiva, who appears in his form as Sadashiva, standing with trident in hand, within a lingam behind the Kundalini Shakti. After this, one should meditate on the Shakti of the chakra, the four-headed Kakini Shakti seated on a lotus flower, who holds in her four hands all the implements needed for acquiring equilibrium. And finally, one should meditate on the Deity of the chakra, Ishana Shiva. The aspirant should visualize the various aspects of each chakra in the particular sequence given above.

Since the duration of the Air element in the breath cycle is only eight minutes, the complete visualization of the Anahata chakra should take place within this time period. Meditation should then take place on the Manipura, Muladhara, Swadhisthana, and Vishuddha chakras respectively. Attention should rest on Manipura chakra

(Fire element) for twelve minutes; the Muladhara chakra (Earth element), twenty minutes; the Swadhishthana chakra (Water element), sixteen minutes; and Vishuddha chakra (Akasha element), four minutes. When, at the end of the Akasha element, the breath starts operating evenly from both nostrils—that is, when the Sushumna begins working—the aspirant should bring his visualization and japa (recitation of seed sounds) to an end and immerse himself in abstract meditation.

For better results in this visualization practice, the aspirant can color drawings of the chakras, in the same order that they should be seen by the inner eye. The order of visualization within each chakra is as follows:

1. Petals (in a clockwise direction)
2. Yantra of the chakra
3. Animal of the chakra
4. Bija sound*
5. Deities other than the presiding deity and the main Shakti
6. Shakti of the chakra
7. Presiding Deity of the chakra

Meditation on the chakras, combined with the performance of one's daily duties in accordance with the energy of the operating nostril, will lead the Swara yogi toward the ultimate goal.

The breath flow, through the left and right nostril, is the same for people of all castes, creeds, and faiths. Although it was discovered by the Tantrics who came from a particular cultural background and who had a language influenced by their unique genetic code, Swara Yoga points toward a Truth which is both universal and fundamental.

*Reciting the bija sound with a nasal resonance (ng), simultaneous to the visualization, brings about a meditative state.

APPENDIX

Extracts from Swara Yoga Scriptures with Commentary by the Author

The scripture Shiva Swarodaya, one of the main sources for the information presented in this work, starts with a dialogue between Shiva and Shakti about the nature of the universe and the knowledge that is essential to live happy, healthy, and inspired lives.

देव देव महादेव कृपां कृत्वा ममोपरि ।
सर्व सिद्ध करं ज्ञानं कथयस्वमम प्रभो ॥

कथं ब्रह्मांडमुत्पन्नं कथं वा परिवर्त्तते ।
कथं विलीयते देव वद ब्रह्मांडनिर्णयम् ॥

Deva deva mahadeva kripam krittva mamopari—
Sarvssiddhi karam gyanam kathyaswa mam prabho—2—
Katham brahmandamutpannam katham va parivartee—
Katham viliyate deva vada bhahmand nirnayam—3—

O Lord of Gods, Mahadev, please be kind to me and tell me about the knowledge that gives all siddhis—the power to achieve whatever one desires.

How has this universe evolved? How does it change from one form to another? Where does it merge during the period of annihilation? Please explain to me the process of creation, preservation, and destruction of this universe.

Listening to this eternal question of his divine consort, Shiva—the Supreme consciousness in male form—said:

तत्त्वाद् ब्रह्मांडमुत्पन्नं तत्त्वेन परिवत्तते।
तत्त्वे विलीयते देवि तत्त्वाद् ब्रह्मांडनिर्णय:॥

Tattvad brahmandamutpannam tattven parivartite—
Tattve viliyate devi tattvad brahmand nirnayah—4—

The universe has originated from the tattvas (the elements). All changes in the world of names and form are changes in the elements; into the elements all merge at the time of annihilation. The elements are, O Devi, the main constituents of this universe.

Hearing the precise answer of Shiva, Shakti asked him to explain the nature of the elements that are important for this manifest world. Shiva said:

निरञ्जनो निराकार एको देव महेश्वर:।
तस्मादाकाशमुत्पन्नमाकाशाद् वायु संमव:॥

वायोस्तेजस्ततश्चापस्ततः पृथ्वी समुद्भव:।
एतानि पंच तत्वानि विस्तीर्णा च पंचधा:॥

Niranjano nirakara eiko dev maheshwarah—
Tasmadakashamutpannamakashad vayu sambhavah—6—
Vayustejastatashchapastatah prithvisamudbhavah—
Aitani panch tattvani visteerna cha panchdha—7—

There was, in the beginning, the one without name
and form; the one without any attributes. From him
originated Akasha; from Akasha originated Air; from Air
originated Fire; from Fire, Water and from Water, Earth.
These five elements then each divided themselves into
five and created the multiple forms of the visible world.

पंचतत्त्वमये देहे पञ्चतत्त्वानि सुन्दरि।
सूक्ष्मरुपेण वर्त्तन्ते ज्ञायन्ते तत्त्वयोगिभि:॥

Panchtattvamaye dehe panchtattvani sundari—
Sukshmroopen vartante gyayante tattvayogibhih—9—

This body is composed of these very five elements.
They form the skin, the flesh, the bones, the marrow, the
nerves, etc. Each and every cell is composed of these
elements. They create the work organs, sense organs,
and the nourishment necessary for the operation of the
different constituents of the body, in gross and subtle
form.

Elements appear and dissolve in their subtle form in
the body and its psychic centers (chakras) in each nasal
cycle, providing nourishment. All desires, feelings, and
emotions are related to these five elements. The elements
are at the root of the psychodrama of life. Only yogis
know this truth.

Yogis know this truth because they are the ones who try to achieve a state of consciousness that is beyond the reach of the elements. Elements cause the mind to fluctuate and make one wander in the forest of desires.

This primary scripture of Swara Yoga, *Shiva Swarodaya,* goes on to praises the science of breath as the highest wisdom. Shiva says:

स्वरे वेदाश्च शास्त्राणि स्वरे गाँधर्वमुत्तमम् ।
स्वरे च सर्वत्रैलोक्यं स्वरमात्मस्वरूपकम् ॥

Sware vedashch shastrani sware gandharvamuttamum—
Sware ch sarvatrailokyam swarmatm—swaroopkam—16—

Swaras are the Vedas and Shastras (the scriptures); swaras are the best music. The matrikas (consonants and vowels) are swaras themselves. In other words, swaras encompass the entire wisdom...the music and sound of the universe.

गुह्यादु गुह्यतरं सारमुपकार प्रकाशनम् ।
इदं स्वरोदयं ज्ञानं ज्ञानानां मस्तके मणिः॥

Guhiyad guihitaram saramupkar prakashnam—
Idam swarodayam gyanam gyananam mastake mahih—11—

This knowledge of the swaras gives access to the secret of all secret sciences, brings forth the essence of all knowledge, and gives awareness. This knowledge of Swara is the crown gem on the head of knowledge.

स्वर हीनश्च देवज्ञो नाथ हीनं यथा गृहम् ।
शास्त्र हीनं यथा वक्त्रं शिरोहीनं च यद्वपुः॥

Swarhinashch devagyo nath hinam yatha graham—
Shastra hinam yatha vaktram shirohinam ch yudwipu—17—

A seer who has no knowlege of the swara is like a barren house, like an orator without authentic knowledge, a body without a head.

अथ स्वरं प्रवक्ष्यामि शरीरस्थस्वरोदयम् ।
हंस चारस्वरूपेण भवेज्ज्ञानं   त्रिकालजम् ॥

Ath swaram pravakshyami sharirasthswarodayam—
Hamschar swaroopena bhavejgyanam trikalajam—10—

Now I will tell you about the swara, which is the main source of true knowledge.

सूक्ष्मात्सूक्ष्मतरं ज्ञानं सुबोधं सत्य प्रत्ययम् ।
आश्चर्यं नास्तिके लोके ह्याधारं त्वास्तिके जने ॥

Sukshmatsukshmataram gyanam subodham satyaprattyam—
Ashcharyam nastike loke hyadharamtwastike jane—12—

Although this knowledge is subtle, it does give a clear understanding of the Truth. It makes one experience the Truth and expands the scope of body/mind coordination. To nonbelievers this knowledge is surprising; to believers it is a great support.

श्रृणु त्वं कथितं देवि देहस्थं   ज्ञानमुत्तमम् ।
यस्य विज्ञान मात्रेण सर्वज्ञत्वं प्रणीयते ॥

Shrun twam kathitam devi behastham gyanamuttamam—
Yasya vigyan matren sarvagyatwam praniyate—15—

Listen O Devi! Now I will tell you the knowledge essential for all who dwell in their body, by knowing which all that which is knowable is known.

नाड़ी भेद तथा प्राणतत्त्व भेदं तथैव च ।
सुषम्णा मिश्रभेदं च यो जानाति समुक्तिग: ॥

Nadibhedam tatha pranatattva bhedam tathaiv cha—
Sushumna mishra bhedam cha yojanati samuktigah—18—

One who knows the secrets of the nadis (their operation and effect), of prana (the difference between the five kinds of prana), and of Sushumna, gets liberated from the cycle of life and death and becomes totally enlightened.

नाड़ी त्रयं विजानाति तत्त्व ज्ञानं तथैव च ।
नैव तेन भवेत्तुल्यं लक्षकोटिरसायनम् ॥

Naditrayam vijanati tattvagyanam tathaiv cha—
Naiv tain bhavettullyam lakshkotirasayanam—29—

One who knows about the three nadis and the five tattvas cannot be equaled with a billion rasayanas (precious medicines that provide nutrients necessary for rejuvenation).

One who has this precious knowledge is unique, because he or she knows the technique of working with the body, mind, and consciousness in the most efficient way.

Doing the right thing at the right moment makes one unique—a genius, whereas doing the right thing at the wrong moment makes one stupid. Those who practice the science of Swara Yoga never suffer from failure and discontent; they know how to change the vibrational pattern of the environment to their advantage.

INDEX

BOOKS OF RELATED INTEREST

Chakras
Energy Centers of Transformation
by Harish Johari

Sounds of the Chakras (CD)
by Harish Johari

Tools for Tantra
by Harish Johari

Sounds of Tantra (CD)
Mantra Meditation Techniques from Tools for Tantra
by Harish Johari

Microchakras
Techniques for InnerTuning
by Sri Shyamji Bhatnagar and David Isaacs, Ph.D.

Secret Power of Tantrik Breathing
Techniques for Attaining Health, Harmony, and Liberation
by Swami Sivapriyananda

The Yoga of the Nine Emotions
The Tantric Practice of Rasa Sadhana
by Peter Marchand
Based on the teachings of Harish Johari

Ways to Better Breathing
by Carola Speads

Inner Traditions • Bear & Company
P.O. Box 388
Rochester, VT 05767
1-800-246-8648
www.InnerTraditions.com

Or contact your local bookseller